POCKET ATLAS OF NORMAL SPINE MRI

Second Edition

Pocket Atlas of Normal Spine MRI

Second Edition

Leo F. Czervionke, MD

Associate Professor
Department of Radiology
Mayo Clinic Jacksonville
Jacksonville, Florida

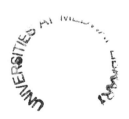

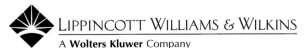

LIPPINCOTT WILLIAMS & WILKINS
A **Wolters Kluwer** Company
Philadelphia • Baltimore • New York • London
Buenos Aires • Hong Kong • Sydney • Tokyo

Acquisitions Editor: Joyce-Rachel John
Developmental Editor: Ellen DiFrancesco
Printer: Sheridan Press

© 2001 by LIPPINCOTT WILLIAMS & WILKINS
530 Walnut Street
Philadelphia, PA 19106 USA
LWW.com

Printed in the USA

Library of Congress Cataloging-in-Publication Data

Czervionke, Leo F.
   Pocket atlas of normal spine MRI/Leo F. Czervionke.—2nd ed.
   p.; cm.
   Includes bibliographical references.
   ISBN-13: 978-0-7817-2948-2
   ISBN-10: 0-7817-2948-3
   1. Spinal cord—Magnetic resonance imaging—Atlases. 2. Spine—Magnetic resonance imaging—Atlases. I. Title
   [DNLM: 1. Spine—anatomy & histology—Atlases. 2. Spine—anatomy & histology—Handbooks. 3. Magnetic Resonance Imaging—Atlases. 4. Magnetic Resonance Imaging—Handbooks. 5. Spinal Cord—anatomy & histology—Atlases. 6. Spinal Cord—anatomy & histology—Handbooks. WE 17 C9977p 2000]
   QM465 .C94 2000
   611'.82'0222—dc21   00-042119

10 9 8 7

Preface

Magnetic resonance imaging of the spine can be deceptively challenging, even to those with a great deal of experience in this area. While the anatomic features of the cervical, thoracic, and lumbosacral spine are in some sense repetitive, unique anatomic features are present in each portion of the spine. An attempt is made to emphasize these features in this book. Clinically relevant sagittal, axial, coronal, and oblique imaging planes were chosen for image representation.

The images selected include 83 high-quality scans of the spine obtained from volunteers and cadaver specimens. Each scan is linked to a localizing image for orientation. Several anatomic images obtained from cadaver cryomicrotome studies are included for correlation in certain key anatomic areas of the spine, and were acquired while on staff at the Medical College of Wisconsin. These MR images were obtained using either a 1.5T General Electric Signa MR scanner (GE Medical Systems, Milwaukee WI) or a 1.5T Siemens Symphony Scanner (Siemens Medical Systems, Erlangen, Germany).

Almost all images for this edition were created with current imaging techniques [e.g., conventional T1 weighted spin echo, gradient echo, and T2 weighted Fast (turbo) spin echo pulse sequences]. Conventional T1 weighted spin echo imaging remains extremely valuable in evaluation of spinal disease. T2 weighted fast spin echo or turbo spin echo are obtained in standard imaging of the spine. These are often obtained with fat suppression techniques in order to render disease processes more conspicuous. Gradient echo images are especially valuable in the cervical region where the epidural venous plexus is prominent and provides inherent contrast to other anatomic structures. Gradient echo images are also useful for evaluating fractures or areas of bone destruction. While not included in this atlas, STIR images provide a valuable adjunct to conventional MR imaging for detection of spinal vertebral disorders.

MR images were obtained from the volunteers with standard imaging parameters. A 256×256 matrix was routinely used with 4mm slice thickness for sagittal images. Oblique, coronal, and axial images were obtained with 3mm slice thickness in the cervical and thoracic spine and 5mm in the lumbar spine. The MR images obtained in the cadaver specimens were quite long (30 to 40 minutes) to enhance visualization of the anatomy such as the gray-white matter differentiation in the spinal cord or ligamentous anatomy.

This updated second edition of the *Pocket Atlas of Spinal MRI* is intended as a practical reference guide to assist physicians and allied health professionals who interpret or perform MR imaging studies of the spine. This edition includes a new section on the occipital-cervical junction with emphasis on the upper cervical ligaments and atlantoaxial articulations. The anatomy of the paraspinal musculature is also stressed in this book.

Acknowledgements

I wish to sincerely thank Lisa Broddle, Lynn Hill, and Kelly Young for their invaluable assistance with the MR imaging of volunteers for this project.

I also wish to gratefully acknowledge my friends and former colleagues David L. Daniels, Victor M. Haughton, Leighton P. Mark, and Alan L. Williams for their generous academic support and consideration during the many years we spent together at the Medical College of Wisconsin.

Special thanks to Jeanne, my wife, who is always there for me.

Contents

Preface v

Cervical Spine 1

Craniocervical Junction 29

Thoracic Spine 43

Thoracolumbar Junction 59

Lumbar Spine 65

Sacrum 95

References 105

POCKET ATLAS OF
NORMAL SPINE MRI

Second Edition

Cervical Spine _____

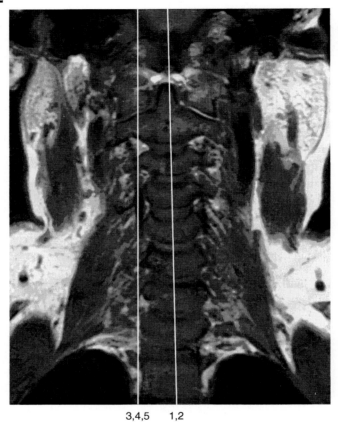

3,4,5   1,2

(L1) Localizer for sagittal cervical spine images.

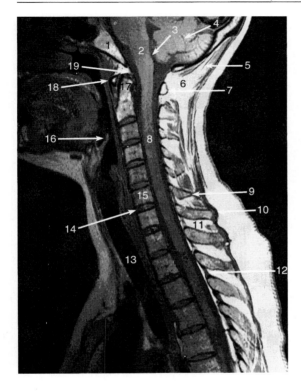

FIG. 1. Midline sagittal T1 spin echo cervical spine: Cervical spinal cord

1. clivus
2. medulla
3. obex
4. cerebellum
5. semispinalis capitis muscle
6. nuchal ligament
7. posterior arch C1
8. cervical spinal cord
9. spinous process C6
10. supraspinous ligament
11. interspinous ligament
12. ligamentum flavum
13. ttacheal airway
14. intervertebral disc C6-7
15. vertebral body C6
16. epiglottis
17. dens (odontoid process)
18. anterior arch C1
19. superior fascicle of cruciform ligament/tectorial membrane

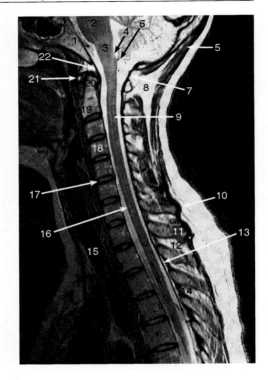

FIG. 2. Midline sagittal T2 fast spin echo cervical spine

1. clivus
2. pons
3. medulla
4. obex
5. semispinalis capitis muscle
6. clava
7. posterior occiptal-atlantal membrane
8. nuchal ligament
9. gray matter along central canal
10. supraspinous ligament
11. spinous process T1
12. interspinous ligament
13. posterior dural sac
14. ligamentum flavum
15. tracheal airway
16. spinal cord
17. intervertebral disc C5-6
18. vertebral body C4
19. vertebral body C2
20. dens (odontoid process)
21. anterior arch C1
22. superior fascicle of cruciform ligament/tectorial membrane

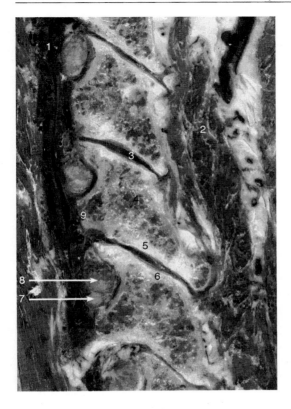

FIG. 3. Parasagittal cadaver cryomicrotome through articular pillar, neural foramen

1. vertebral artery
2. multifidis muscle
3. apophyseal (facet) joint
4. articular pillar
5. inferior articular process
6. superior articular process
7. ventral root (motor)
8. dorsal root ganglion
9. pedicle

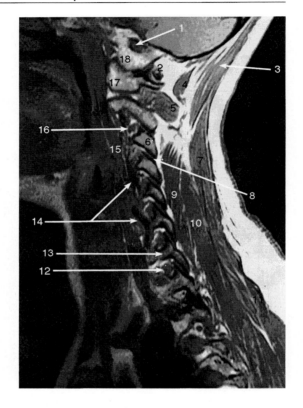

FIG. 4. Parasagittal T1 spin echo neural foramen

1. hypoglossal canal
2. vertebral artery
3. semispinalis capitis muscle
4. rectus capitis posterior major muscle
5. obliquus capitis inferior muscle
6. articular pillar C3
7. splenius capitis muscle
8. apophyseal (facet) joint C3-4
9. multifidis muscle
10. semispinalis cervicis muscle
11. trapezius muscle
12. C8 dorsal root ganglion
13. C7 pedicle
14. vertebral artery
15. longus colli (cervicis) muscle
16. C3 dorsal root ganglion
17. lateral mass C1
18. occipital condyle

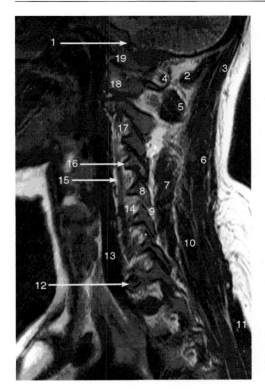

FIG. 5. Parasagittal T2 fast spin echo: Cervical neural foramen, vertebral artery

1. hypoglossal canal
2. rectus capitis posterior major muscle
3. semispinalis capitis muscle
4. vertebral artery
5. obliquus capitis inferior muscle
6. splenius capitis muscle
7. multifidis muscle
8. articular pillar
9. apophyseal (facet) joint C5-6
10. semispinalis cervicis muscle
11. trapezius muscle
12. head of 1st rib
13. longus colli (cervicis) muscle
14. dorsal root ganglion C6
15. vertebral artery
16. pedicle C4
17. dorsal root ganglion C3
18. lateral mass C1
19. occipital condyle

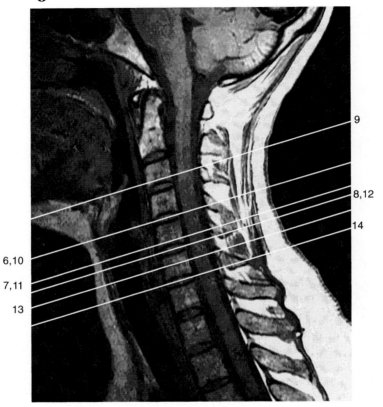

(L2) Localizer for axial images of cervical spine.

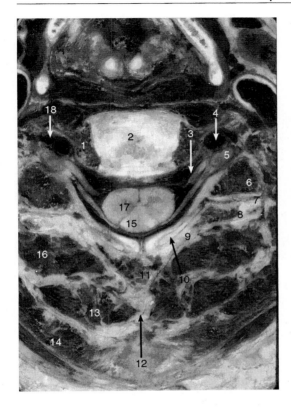

FIG. 6. Axial cadaver anatomic section: C4-5 level

1. uncinate process
2. intervertebral disc
3. ventral rootlet bundle C6
4. vertebral artery
5. dorsal root ganglion C6
6. superior articular process C6
7. apophyseal (facet) joint
8. inferior articular process C5
9. lamina C5
10. ligamentum flavum
11. spinous process C5
12. ligamentum nuchae
13. semispinalis capitis muscle
14. splenius capitis muscle
15. dorsal white matter column
16. multifidis and semispinalis cervicis muscles
17. ventral horn gray matter
18. paravertebral vein

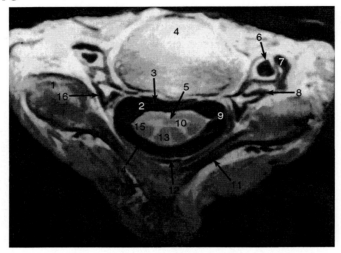

FIG. 7. Axial T1 spin echo in cadaver: Superior neural foramen C5-6 level

1. superior articular process C6
2. ventral rootlet
3. anterior dura of thecal sac
4. C5 vertebral body
5. ventral white matter column (funiculus)
6. vertebral artery
7. paravertebral vein
8. foraminal veins
9. dentate ligament
10. gray matter of spinal cord
11. lamina
12. posterior dura of thecal sac
13. posterior white matter column (funiculus)
14. dorsal rootlet
15. lateral white matter column (funiculus)
16. foraminal veins

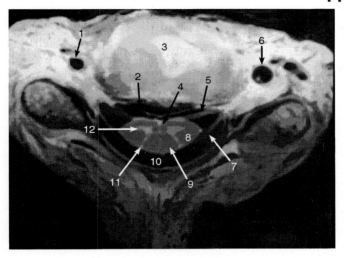

FIG 8. Axial T1 spin echo cadaver: Lower foramen C5-6 level

1. right vertebral artery
2. anterior dura of thecal sac
3. intervertebral disc C5-6
4. anterior funiculus
5. ventral rootlet C6
6. left vertebral artery
7. dorsal rootlet C6
8. lateral funiculus
9. dorsal funiculus
10. subarachnoid space
11. dorsal gray matter horn
12. ventral gray matter horn

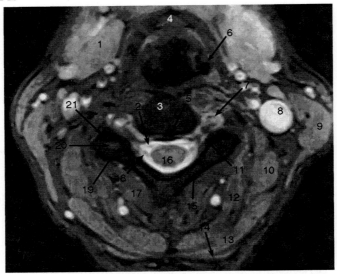

FIG. 9. Axial gradient echo: Superior neural foramen C3-4 level

1. submandibular gland
2. ventral rootlet
3. C3 vertebral body
4. hyoid bone
5. posterior longitudinal ligament/anterior thecal sac dura
6. pyriform sinus
7. vertebral artery
8. internal jugular vein
9. sternocleidomastoid muscle
10. longissimus capitis muscle
11. neural foramen, nerve root sheath
12. semispinalis capitis muscle
13. splenius capitis muscle
14. trapezius muscle
15. lamina C3
16. dorsal white matter column, spinal cord
17. multifidis muscle
18. dorsal rootlet
19. inferior articular process C3
20. facet joint
21. superior articular process C4

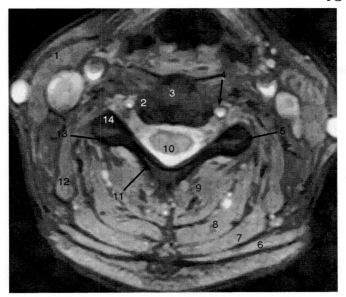

FIG. 10. Axial gradient echo C4-5 foramen level
1. sternocleidomastoid muscle
2. uncinate process
3. intervertebral disc
4. left vertebral artery
5. facet joint C4-5
6. trapezius muscle
7. splenius capitis muscle
8. semispinalis capitis muscle
9. multifidis muscle
10. spinal cord posterior funiculus
11. lamina C3
12. longissimus capitis muscle
13. inferior articular process C3
14. superior articular process C4

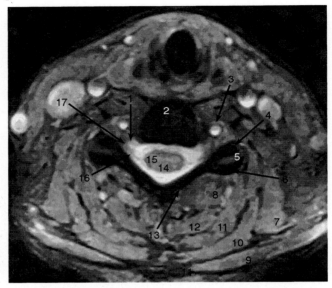

FIG. 11. Axial gradient echo C5-6 upper neural foramen
1. ventral rootlet bundle
2. vertebral body C5
3. vertebral artery
4. superior articular process C6
5. facet (apophyseal) joint C5-6
6. inferior articular process C5
7. levator scapula muscle
8. multifidis muscle
9. trapezius muscle
10. splenius capitis muscle
11. semispinalis capitis muscle
12. semispinalis cervicis muscle
13. lamina C5
14. posterior white matter funiculus, spinal cord
15. gray matter, spinal cord
16. dorsal rootlet bundle
17. dorsal root ganglion C6

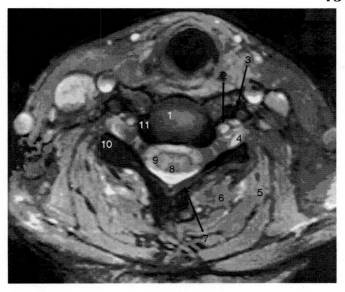

FIG. 12. Axial gradient echo C5-6 disc level
1. intervertebral disc C5-6
2. vertebral artery
3. lateral mass
4. dorsal root ganglion C6
5. longissimus cervicis muscle
6. multifidis muscle
7. ligamentum flavum
8. spinal cord posterior white matter column
9. spinal cord lateral white matter column
10. superior articular process C6
11. uncinate process C6

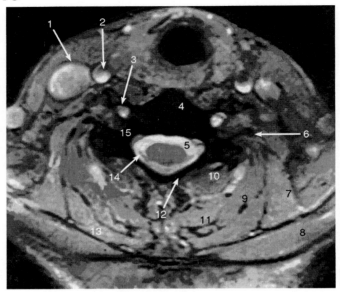

FIG. 13. Axial gradient echo C6 level
1. internal jugular vein
2. common carotid artery
3. vertebral artery
4. vertebral body C6
5. ventral rootlet
6. transverse process
7. levator scapula muscle
8. trapezius muscle
9. semispinalis capitis muscle
10. multifidis muscle
11. semispinalis cervicis muscle
12. lamina C6
13. splenius capitis muscle
14. dorsal rootlet
15. pedicle C6

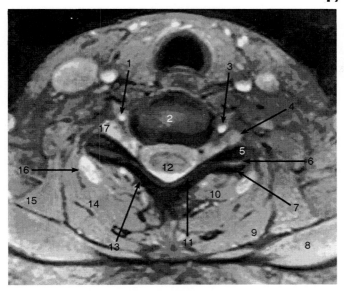

FIG. 14. Axial gradient echo C6-7 disc level
1. right vertebral artery
2. intervertebral disc C6-7
3. left Vertebral artery
4. left dorsal root ganglion C7
5. superior articular process C7
6. facet joint
7. inferior articular process C6
8. trapezius muscle
9. splenius capitis muscle
10. multifidis muscle
11. ligamentum flavum
12. spinal cord posterior white matter column
13. lamina C6
14. semispinalis capitis muscle
15. levator scapula muscle
16. deep cervical vein
17. right dorsal root ganglion C7

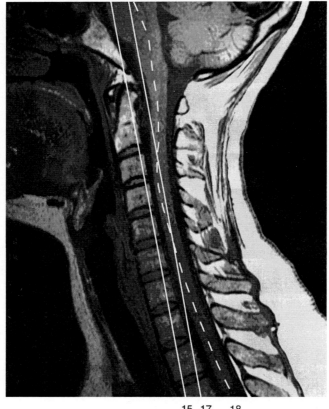

15 17   18
16

(L3) Localizer for coronal cervical spine images.

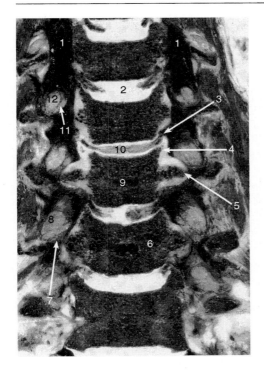

FIG. 15. Coronal cadaver anatomic section through cervical vertebral bodies, neural foramen

1. vertebral artery
2. intervertebral disc
3. uncovertebral joint of Lushka
4. uncinate process
5. pedicle
6. vertebral body
7. ventral nerve root
8. dorsal root ganglion
9. basivertebral vein
10. degenerating intervertebral disc
11. ventral nerve root
12. dorsal root ganglion

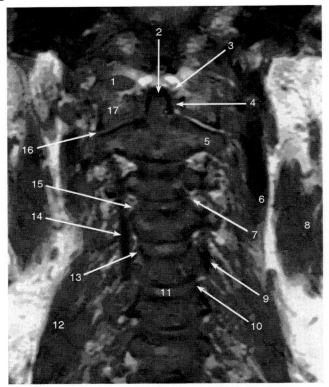

FIG. 16. Coronal T1 spin echo cervical spine

1. occipital condyle
2. dens (odontoid process)
3. alar ligament
4. transverse ligament of dens, lateral portion
5. lateral mass (pillar) C2
6. internal jugular vein
7. left nerve root C4 in neural foramen
8. sternocleidomastoid muscle
9. left vertebral artery
10. uncovertebral joint of Luschka
11. C5-6 intervertebral disc
12. scalene muscle group
13. uncinate process C5
14. right vertebral artery
15. right nerve root C4
16. C1-2 facet joint (lateral atlantoaxial joint)
17. lateral mass C1

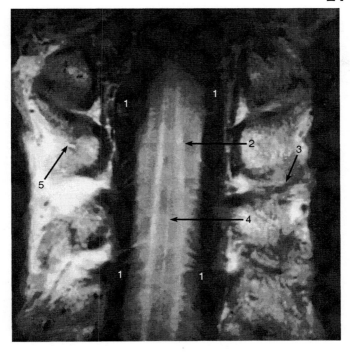

FIG. 17. Coronal T1 spin echo cadaver: Cord gray matter
1. nerve rootlets
2. gray matter, ventral horn
3. facet (apophyseal) joint
4. gray matter along central canal
5. articular pillar

Cervical Spine

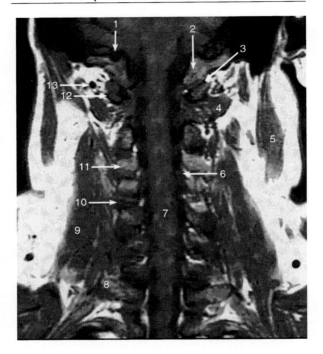

FIG. 18. Coronal T1 spin echo cervical cord

1. hypoglossal canal
2. occipital condyle
3. atlanto-occipital joint
4. obliquus capitis inferior muscle
5. sternocleidomastoid muscle
6. nerve rootlet bundle C4
7. spinal cord
8. transverse process T1
9. scalene muscle group
10. facet joint C4-5
11. articular pillar C4
12. lateral mass C1
13. vertebral artery

19, 20, 21

22, 23

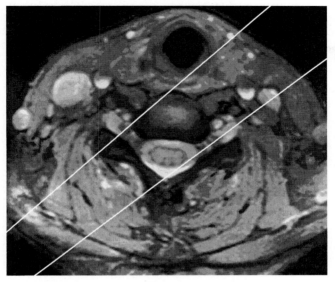

(L4) Localizer for oblique cervical foraminal images.

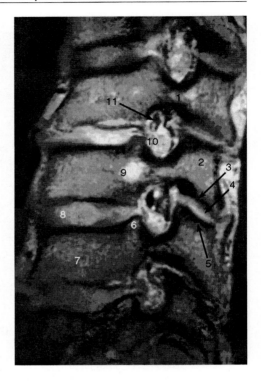

FIG. 19. 45 degree sagittal/coronal T1 SE cadaver: Cervical neural foramen cross section

1. pedicle
2. articular pillar
3. inferior articular process
4. apophyseal (facet) joint
5. superior articular process
6. uncinate process
7. vertebral body
8. intervertebral disc
9. focal fat deposit in vertebral body
10. nerve root in foramen inferiorly
11. superior foraminal veins

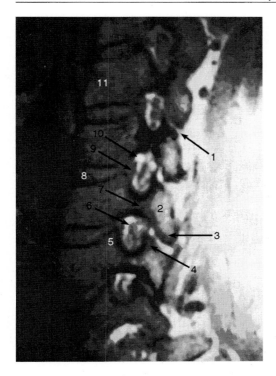

FIG. 20.   45 degree oblique sagittal/coronal T1 spin echo image

1. facet (apophyseal joint)
2. articular pillar
3. inferior articular process
4. superior articular process
5. uncinate process
6. superior foraminal vein
7. pedicle
8. intervertebral disc
9. bulging disc
10. superior foraminal fat
11. vertebral body

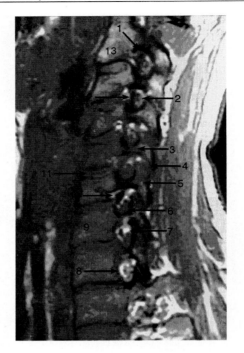

FIG. 21. Curved reformatted 45 degree oblique sagittal T1 spin echo

1. neural foramen C2-3
2. nerve root C4
3. pedicle C5
4. facet joint C5-6
5. articular pillar C6
6. nerve root C7
7. superior foraminal fat
8. neural foramen T1-2
9. vertebral body C7
10. superior foraminal vein
11. intervertebral disc C5-6
12. vertebral artery (volume averaged)
13. vertebral body C2

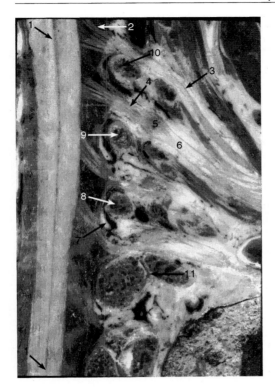

FIG. 22. Sagittal cadaver anatomic section 45 degree oblique, parallel to exiting nerve roots

1. gray matter along central canal of spinal cord
2. nerve rootlets with root pouch
3. C5 nerve root
4. C6 rootlet bundle
5. C6 dorsal root ganglion
6. C6 nerve root
7. foraminal vein
8. pedicle C7
9. pedicle C6
10. pedicle C5
11. 1st costo-transverse joint

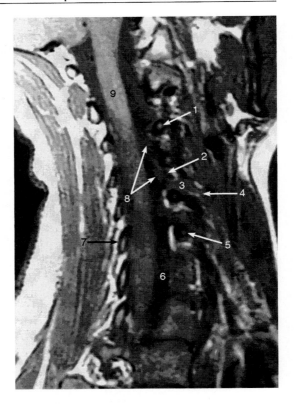

**FIG 23. 45 degree sagittal/coronal oblique T1 spin echo parallel
to exiting left nerve roots**

1. pedicle C3
2. superior foraminal vein
3. dorsal root ganglion C5
4. nerve root C5
5. pedicle C6
6. subarachnoid space
7. lamina C6
8. nerve rootlets within thecal
   sac, C4 and C5
9. spinal cord

Craniocervical Junction

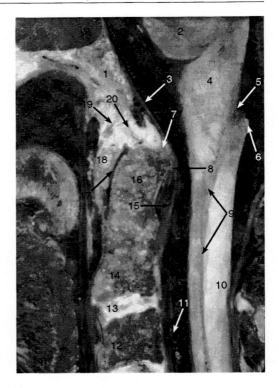

FIG. 24. Midsagittal cervical-medullary junction. Cadaver anatomic section

1. clivus
2. pons
3. tectoral membrane
4. medulla
5. obex
6. clava
7. superior fascicle of cruciform ligament
8. transverse ligament of cruciform ligament
9. gray matter along central canal
10. spinal cord
11. posterior longitudinal ligament
12. C3 vertebral body
13. C2-3 intervertebral disc
14. C2 vertebral body
15. inferior fascicle of cruciform ligament
16. dens
17. anterior atlanto-axial joint
18. anterior arch of C1
19. anterior atalanto-occipital membrane
20. apical ligament of dens

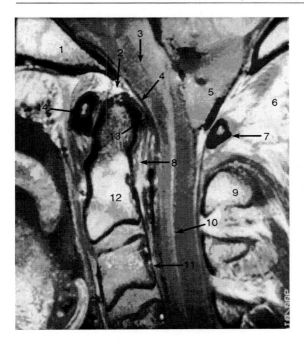

FIG. 25. Sagittal T1 Spin echo cervical-medullary junction, cadaver

1. clivus
2. apical ligament
3. medulla
4. tectorial membrane
5. cerebellar tonsil
6. nuchal ligament
7. posterior arch C1
8. inferior fascicle of cruciform ligament
9. C2 spinous process
10. gray matter along central canal
11. posterior longitudinal ligament
12. C2 vertebral body
13. transverse ligament
14. anterior arch C1

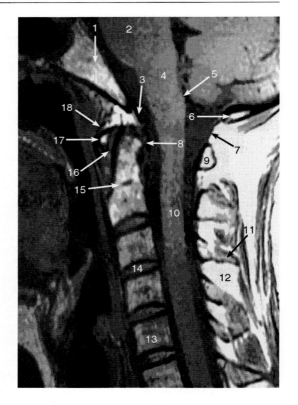

FIG. 26. Midline sagittal T1 spin echo craniocervical junction

1. clivus
2. pons
3. tectorial membrane/superior fascicle cruciform ligament
4. medulla
5. clava
6. occipital bone, posterior lip of foramen magnum
7. posterior atlanto-occipital membrane
8. transverse ligament of cruciform ligament
9. posterior arch C1
10. spinal cord
11. spinous process C3
12. interspinous ligament
13. vertebral body C5
14. intervertebral disc C3-4
15. dental synchondrosis (disc anlage)
16. anterior atlantoaxial joint
17. tubercle anterior arch C1
18. anterior atlanto-occipital membrane

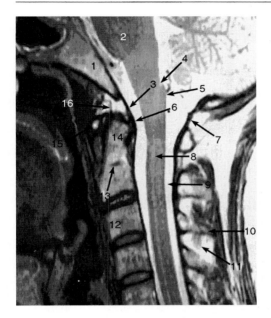

FIG. 27. Midline sagittal T2 fast spin echo occipital-cervical junction

1. clivus
2. pons
3. tectorial membrane/superior fascicle cruciform ligament
4. obex
5. clava
6. transverse ligament of cruciform ligament
7. posterior atlanto-occipital membrane
8. gray matter along central canal
9. subarachnoid space
10. spinous process C3
11. interspinous ligament
12. vertebra body C3
13. dental synchondrosis (C1-2 disc anlage)
14. dens
15. tubercle anterior arch C1
16. apical ligament of dens

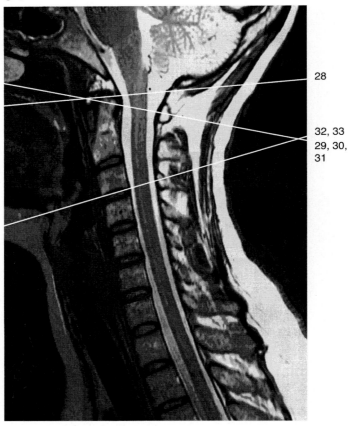

28

32, 33
29, 30,
31

(L5) Localizer for axial images of cervical ligaments.

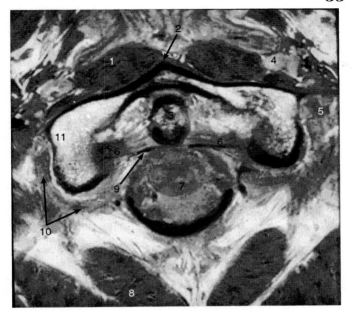

FIG. 28. Axial T1 SE cadaver: High dens level
 1. longus capitis muscle
 2. anterior arch C1
 3. dens
 4. internal carotid artery
 5. vertebral artery exiting transverse foramen
 6. alar ligament
 7. spinal cord
 8. rectus capitis posterior major muscle
 9. tectorial membrane
10. vertebral artery
11. lateral mass C1, superiorly

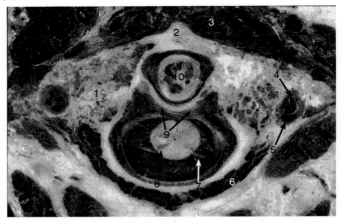

FIG. 29. Axial cadaver anatomic specimen at C1 level
1. lateral mass C1
2. tubercle, anterior arch C1
3. longus capitis muscle
4. Vertebral artery
5. paravertebral vein
6. lamina C1, marrow
7. posterior rootlet
8. dorsal horn, gray matter
9. transverse ligament (part of cruciform ligament)
10. dens (odontoid process)

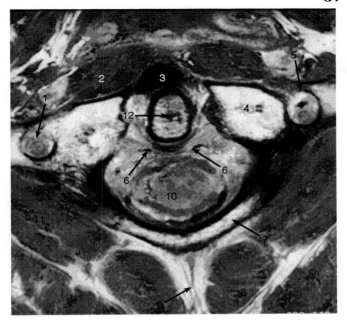

FIG. 30. Axial T1 SE cadaver specimen: Mid-dens level
1. vertebral artery
2. longus capitis muscle
3. anterior arch C1, tubercle
4. lateral mass
5. transverse foramen
6. transverse ligament of cruciform ligament
7. lamina (posterior arch) of C1
8. rectus capitis posterior major muscle
9. nuchal ligament
10. spinal cord
11. obliquus capitis inferior muscle
12. dens (odontoid process)

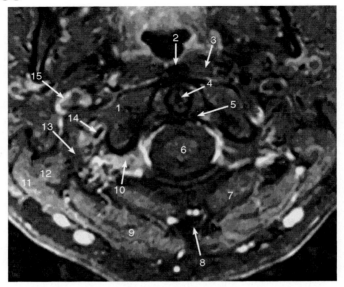

FIG. 31. Axial contrast-enhanced T1 SE, cadaver: Odontoid process, transverse ligament

1. lateral mass C1
2. anterior tubercle C1
3. longus capitis muscle
4. dens (odontoid process)
5. transverse ligament of cruciform ligament
6. spinal cord
7. rectus capitis posterior major muscle
8. nuchal ligament
9. semispinalis capitis muscle
10. C1-2 neural foramen
11. splenius capitis muscle
12. longissimus capitis muscle
13. obliquus capitis inferior muscle
14. vertebral artery
15. internal jugular vein

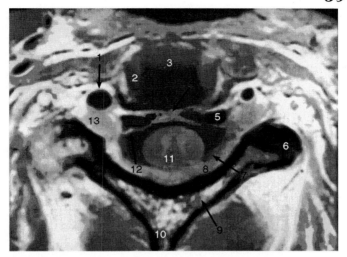

**FIG. 32. Axial T1 SE cadaver. C3-4 intervertebral disc:
Inferior neural foramen, posterior longitudinal ligament**

1. vertebral artery
2. uncinate process
3. intervertebral disc
4. posterior longitudinal ligament
5. anterior epidural vein
6. facet joint
7. dorsal rootlet
8. ligamentum flavum
9. lamina
10. spinous process
11. spinal cord, posterior white matter column
12. anterior thecal sac dura
13. dorsal root ganglion

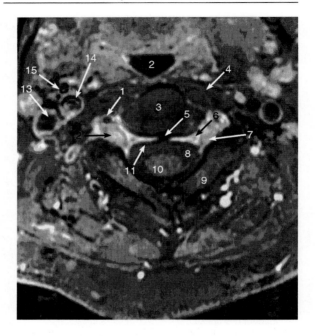

FIG. 33. Axial contrast enhanced T1 spin echo C3-4 foramen
1. vertebral artery
2. airway
3. C3 vertebral body
4. longus colli (longus cervicis) muscle
5. posterior longitudinal ligament, midline portion
6. anterior epidural veins
7. dorsal root ganglion C4
8. subarachnoid space
9. lamina
10. spinal cord
11. dural thecal sac, anterior portion
12. dorsal root ganglion C4
13. internal jugular vein
14. internal carotid artery
15. external carotid artery

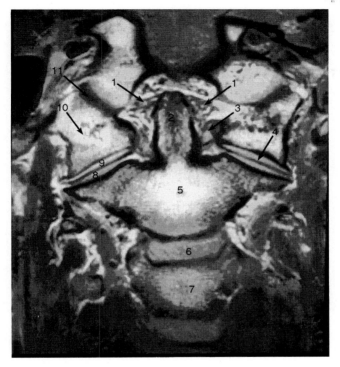

FIG. 34. Coronal T1 spin echo through dens in cadaver
1. alar ligaments
2. dens (odontoid process)
3. transverse ligament, lateral aspect
4. C2-3 facet joint
5. C2 vertebral body
6. C2-3 intervertebral disc
7. C3 vertebral body
8. superior articular cartilage C2
9. inferior articular cartilage C1
10. lateral mass C1
11. atlanto-occipital joint

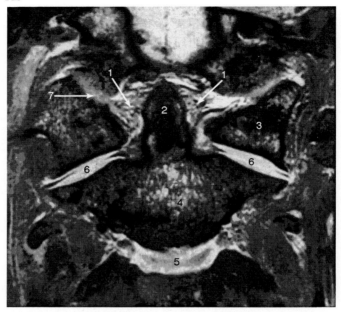

FIG. 35. Coronal T2 gradient echo of C2 in cadaver
1. alar ligaments
2. dens
3. lateral mass C2
4. body of C2
5. C2-3 intervertebral disc
6. facet joints, cartilaginous articulations
7. atlanto-occipital joint

Thoracic Spine _____

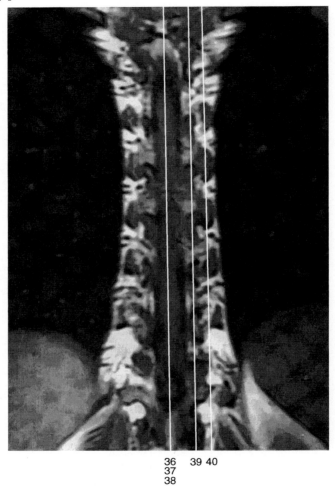

36   39 40
37
38

(L6) Localizer for sagittal thoracic spine images.

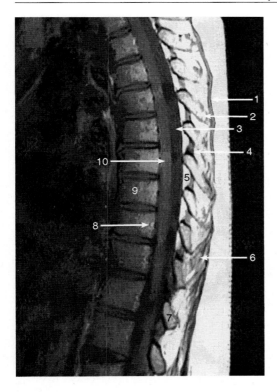

FIG. 36. Midsagittal T1 spin echo: Thoracic spinal cord
1. supraspinous ligament
2. spinous process
3. subarachnoid space
4. ligamentum flavum
5. posterior epidural fat
6. multifidis muscle
7. spinous process
8. basivertebral vein
9. vertebral body
10. spinal cord

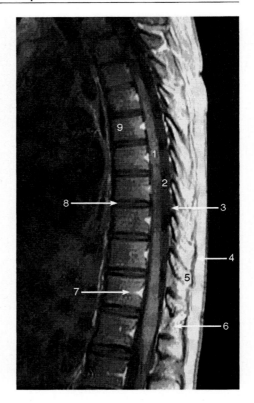

FIG. 37. Midsagittal contrast-enhanced T1 spin echo
1. spinal cord
2. subarachnoid space
3. ligamentum flavum
4. supraspinous ligament
5. spinous process
6. interspinous ligament
7. basivertebral vein
8. intervertebral disc
9. vertebral body

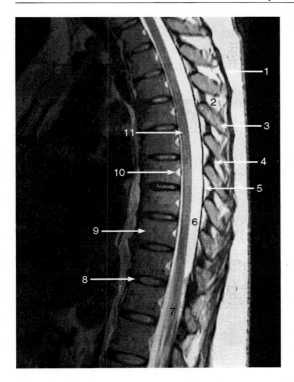

FIG. 38. Midsagittal T2 fast spin echo: Thoracic spinal cord
1. supraspinous ligament
2. interspinous ligament
3. spinous process
4. ligamentum flavum
5. posterior thecal sac dura
6. subarachnoid space
7. conus medullaris
8. intervertebral disc
9. vertebral body
10. basivertebral vein
11. spinal cord

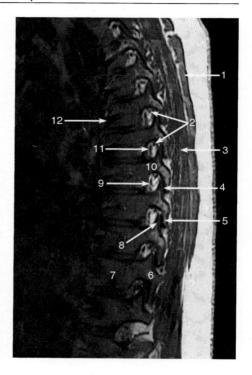

FIG. 39. Parasagittal T1 spin echo: Thoracic neural foramen
1. trapezius muscle
2. foraminal nerve roots
3. erector spinae muscle group
4. facet joint
5. inferior articular process
6. pars interarticularis
7. vertebral body
8. superior articular process
9. foraminal veins
10. pedicle
11. foraminal veins
12. thoracic paravertebral intercostal vein and artery

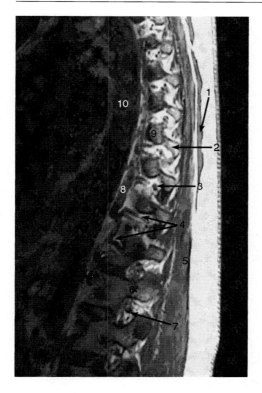

FIG. 40. Parasagittal T1 spin echo: Left paraspinal area
1. trapezius muscle
2. transverse process
3. dorsal root ganglion
4. intercostal veins, paravertebral portions
5. erector spinae muscle group (mainly longissimus dorsi muscle)
6. pedicle
7. nerve root
8. hemiazygous vein
9. head of rib
10. thoracic aorta

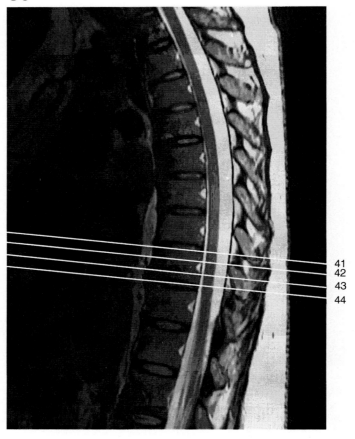

41
42
43
44

(L7) Localizer for axial thoracic spine images.

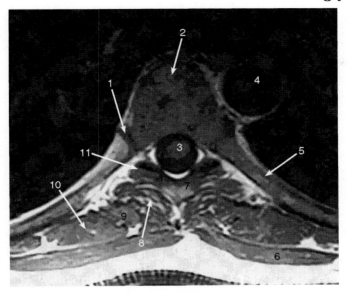

**FIG. 41. Axial T1 spin echo: T9 vertebral body/
costovertebral joint**
 1. costovertebral joint
 2. vertebral body/superior endplate
 3. spinal cord
 4. thoracic aorta
 5. 9th rib
 6. trapezius muscle
 7. lamina
 8. multifidis muscle
 9. spinalis dorsi muscle
10. longissimus dorsi muscle
11. facet joint T8-9

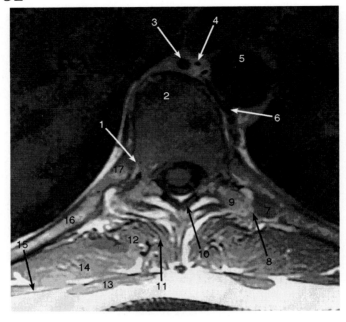

FIG. 42. Axial T1 spin echo: T9 pedicle level

1. costotransverse joint
2. vertebral body
3. azygous vein
4. thoracic duct
5. thoracic aorta
6. intercostal vein joins hemiazygous vein
7. tubercle of left 9th rib
8. costotransverse joint
9. transverse process
10. ligamentum flavum
11. multifidis muscle
12. spinalis dorsi muscle
13. trapezius muscle
14. longissimus dorsi muscle
15. latissimus dorsi muscle
16. right 9th rib
17. head of right 9th rib

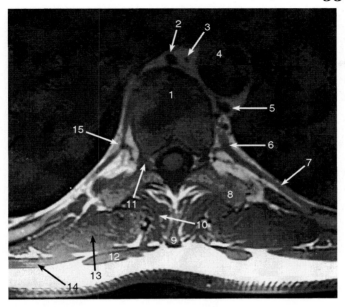

FIG. 43. Axial T1 spin echo: Upper neural foramen T9-10 level
1. vertebra body T9
2. azygous vein
3. thoracic duct
4. aorta
5. hemiazygous vein
6. thoracic paravertebral vein
7. thoracic T9 intercostal vein
8. transverse process T9
9. spinous process
10. multifidis muscle
11. neural foramen/nerve root
12. trapezius muscle
13. longissimus dorsi muscle
14. latissimus dorsi muscle
15. parvertebral veins

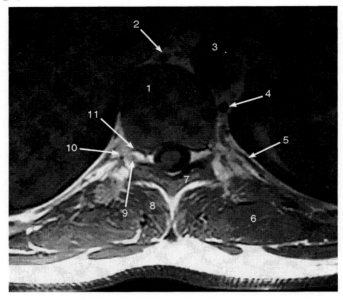

FIG. 44. Axial T1 spin echo: Lower foramen T9-10
1. inferior endplate T9/T9-10 disc
2. azygous vein
3. aorta
4. hemiazygous vein
5. T9 intercostal vein
6. longissimus dorsi muscle
7. lamina
8. multifidis muscle
9. dorsal root ganglion T9
10. paravertebral venous plexus
11. anterior foraminal vein

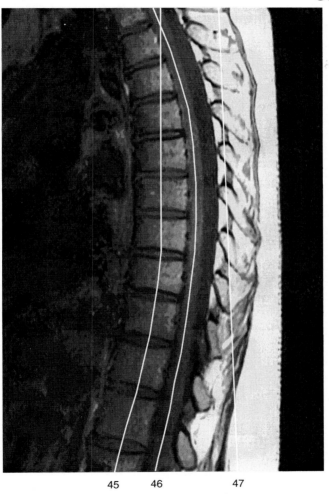

45   46   47

(L8) Localizer for coronal thoracic spine images.

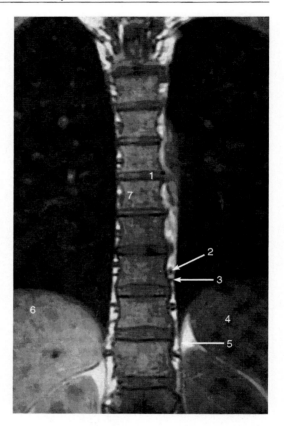

FIG. 45. Coronal curved reformatted T1 spin echo: Thoracic vertebral bodies
1. intervertebral disc
2. intercostal vein
3. intercostal artery
4. spleen
5. left diaphragmatic crus
6. liver
7. vertebral body

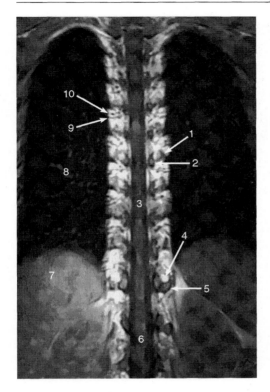

FIG. 46. Coronal curved reformatted T1 spin echo: Thoracic spinal canal
1. head of rib
2. pedicle
3. spinal cord
4. costovertebral joint
5. head of rib
6. conus medullaris
7. liver
8. right lung
9. intercostal artery
10. intercostal vein

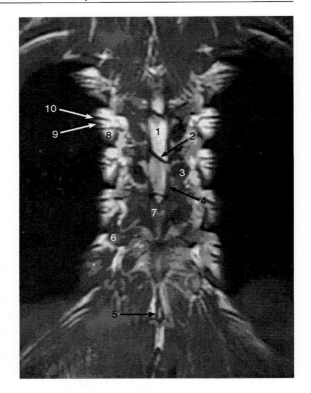

FIG. 47. Coronal T1 spin echo: Ligamentum flavum, thoracic facets
1. posterior epidural fat
2. posterior epidural vein
3. facets/facet joint
4. ligamentum flavum
5. spinous process
6. transverse process
7. lamina
8. head of rib
9. intercostal artery
10. intercostal vein

Thoracolumbar Junction

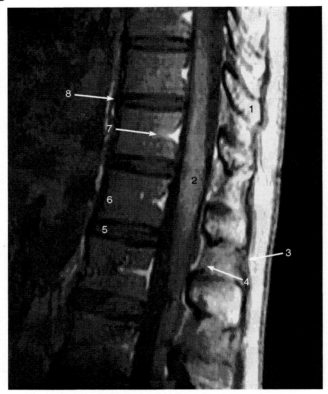

FIG. 48. Contrast-enhanced midsagittal T1 spin echo: Conus medullaris
1. spinous process
2. conus medullaris
3. supraspinous ligament
4. ligamentum flavum
5. intervertebral disc
6. vertebral body
7. basivertebral vein enhancing
8. anterior longitudinal ligament

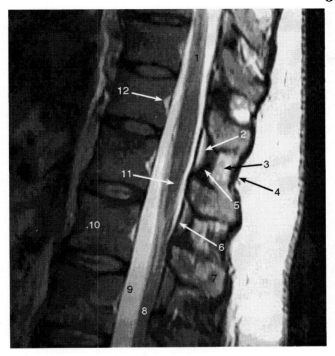

FIG. 49. Midsagittal T2 fast spin echo: Conus medullaris
 1. spinal cord
 2. posterior epidural fat
 3. interspinous ligament
 4. supraspinous ligament
 5. ligamentum flavum
 6. posterior dura/chemical shift
 7. spinous process
 8. cauda equina nerve rootlets
 9. subarachnoid space
10. vertebral body
11. conus medullaris
12. basivertebral vein

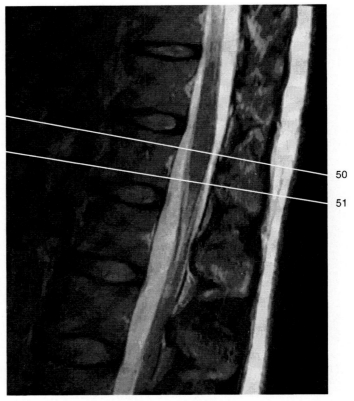

50

51

(L9) Localizer for axial conus images.

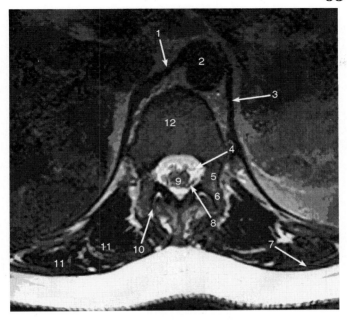

FIG. 50. Axial T2 fast spin echo: Conus medullaris/low spinal cord

1. right diaphragmatic crus
2. abdominal aorta
3. left diaphragmatic crus
4. ventral rootlet
5. pedicle
6. superior articular process
7. latissimus dorsi muscle
8. dorsal rootlet
9. conus medullaris
10. facet joint
11. erector spinae muscle group
12. vertebral body

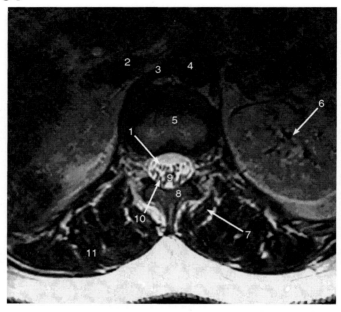

FIG. 51. Axial T2 fast spin echo: Conus medullaris tip
1. ventral rootlets
2. inferior vena cava
3. right diaphramgatic crus
4. aorta
5. intervertebral disc
6. kidney
7. multifidis muscle
8. lamina
9. conus medullaris tip
10. dorsal rootlets
11. erector spinae muscle group

Lumbar Spine _____

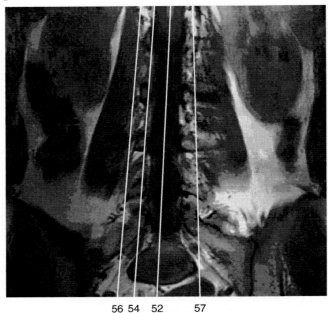

56 54 52   57
   55 53

(L10) Localizer for sagittal lumbar spine images.

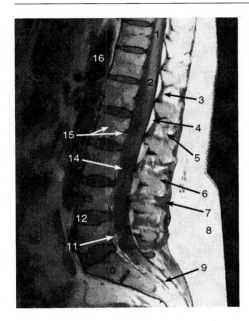

FIG. 52. Midsagittal T1 spin echo: Lumbar spinal canal
 1. spinal cord
 2. conus medullaris
 3. ligamentum flavum
 4. posterior epidural fat
 5. interspinous ligament and Interspinalis lumborum muscle
 6. spinous process
 7. supraspinous ligament
 8. subcutaneous fat
 9. caudal dura/filum terminale
10. S1 vertebral body
11. anterior epidural venous plexus
12. intervertebral disc
13. vertebra body L4
14. subarachnoid space
15. basivertebral venous plexus
16. abdominal aorta

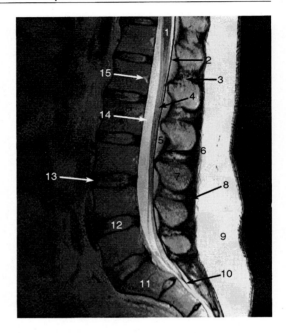

FIG. 53. Midsagittal T2 fast spin echo: Lumbar spinal canal
1. conus medullaris
2. posterior dura of thecal sac
3. interspinous ligament
4. cauda equina
5. posterior epidural fat
6. ligamentum flavum
7. spinous process L3
8. supraspinous ligament
9. subcutaneous fat
10. caudal dura of thecal sac/filum terminale
11. S1 vertebral body
12. intervertebral disc nucleus pulposus L4-5
13. outer annulus L3-4 intervertebral disc
14. subarachnoid space
15. basivertebral vein

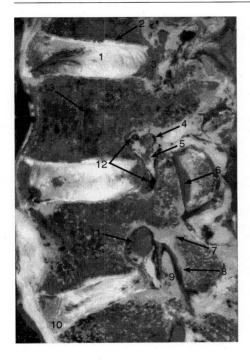

FIG. 54. Parasagittal cadaver anatomic section: Lumbar neural foramen
1. nucleus pulposus
2. vertebral endplate
3. posterior disc annulus
4. dorsal root ganglion
5. ventral rootlet bundle
6. apophyseal (facet) joint
7. pars interarticularis
8. inferior articular process
9. superior articular process
10. anterior disc annulus
11. dorsal root ganglion
12. superior and inferior foraminal veins
13. vertebral body centrum

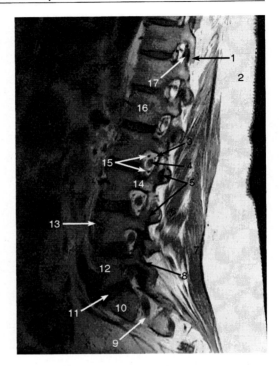

FIG. 55. Parasagittal T1 spin echo: Lumbar neural foramen
1. inferior articular process
2. subcutaneous fat
3. superior foraminal vein
4. dorsal root ganglion
5. facet joint
6. multifidis muscle
7. erector spinae muscle group
8. pars interarticularis
9. S1 nerve root in 1st sacral neural foramen
10. S1 vertebral body
11. L5-S1 intervertebral disc
12. L5 vertebral body
13. lumbar vein
14. pedicle
15. superior and inferior foraminal veins
16. vertebral body
17. superior articular process

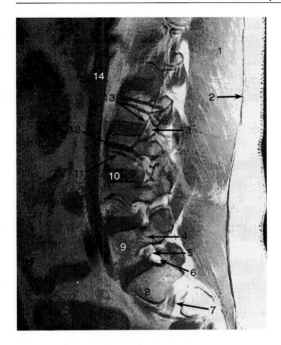

FIG. 56. Parasagittal T1 spin echo: Paravertebral veins
 1. erector spinae muscle group
 2. thoracolumbar fascia, posterior layer
 3. L2 dorsal root ganglion
 4. pedicle L5
 5. L5 root ganglion
 6. foraminal fat
 7. S1 nerve root in 1st sacral foramen
 8. S1 vertebral body
 9. L5 vertebra body
 10. L3-4 intervertebral disc
 11. L3 lumbar artery
 12. L3 lumbar vein
 13. longitudinal (vertical) vein
 14. inferior vena cava

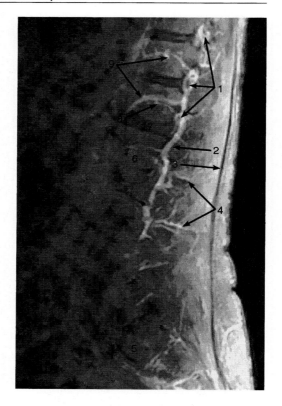

FIG. 57. Contrast-enhanced paravertebral veins
1. nerve roots surrounded be foraminal venous plexus
2. longitudinal (vertical) vein
3. thoracolumbar fascia, posterior portion
4. posterior paraspinal veins
5. S1 vertebral body
6. L2 vertebral body
7. L1-2 intervertebral disc
8. L1 lumbar artery
9. lumbar veins, T12 and L1

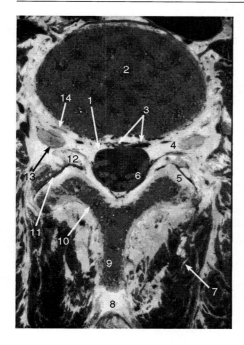

FIG. 58. Axial cadaver anatomic section L4 vertebral body: Upper neural foramen level

1. thecal sac
2. vertebral body centrum
3. anterior epidural veins
4. fat in neural foramen
5. inferior articular process L4
6. nerve rootlets of cauda equina
7. multifidis muscle
8. supraspinous ligament
9. spinous process L4
10. lamina L4
11. facet joint
12. ligamentum flavum (yellow ligament)
13. dorsal root ganglion
14. ventral root

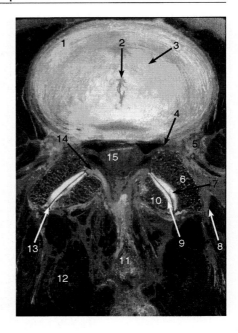

FIG. 59. Axial cadaver anatomic section L3-4 disc level
1. outer annulus
2. nucleus pulposus
3. inner annulus
4. nerve rootlet bundle
5. dorsal root ganglion in neural foramen
6. superior articular process of L4
7. articular cartilage of superior articular facet L3
8. dorsal ramus of L3 nerve
9. articular cartilage of inferior articular facet L3
10. inferior articular process of L3
11. spinous process
12. multifidis muscle
13. facet joint
14. ligamentum flavum
15. nerve rootlets of cauda equina in thecal sac

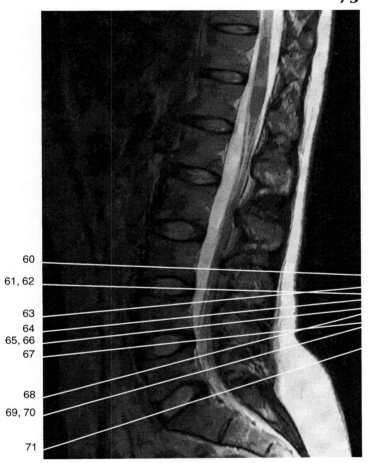

60
61, 62
63
64
65, 66
67
68
69, 70
71

(L11) Localizer for axial lumbar spine images.

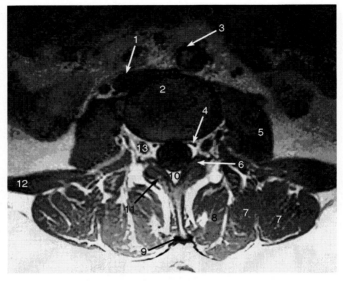

FIG. 60. Axial T1 spin echo: L3 vertebral body/upper L3-4 neural foramen level

1. inferior vena cava
2. L3 vertebral body
3. infrarenal abdominal aorta
4. anterior epidural vein
5. psoas muscle
6. ligamentum flavum
7. erector spinae muscle group
8. multifidis muscle
9. spinous process
10. posterior epidural fat
11. lamina L3
12. quadratus lumborum muscle
13. dorsal root ganglion L3

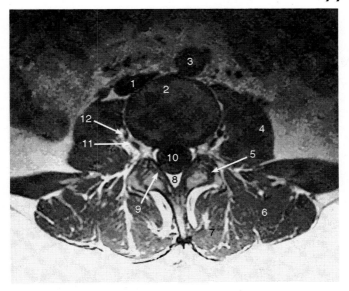

FIG. 61. Axial T1 spin echo: Low L3-4 neural foramen level
1. inferior vena cava
2. L3-4 intervertebral disc
3. abdominal aorta
4. psoas muscle
5. L3-4 facet joint
6. erector spinae muscle group
7. multifidis muscle
8. posterior epidural fat
9. ligamentum flavum
10. subarachnoid space in thecal sac
11. L3 nerve root
12. paravertebral longitudinal vein

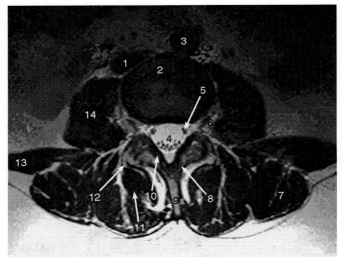

FIG. 62. Axial T1 spin echo: Low L3-4 neural foramen level
1. inferior vena cava
2. L3-4 intervertebral disc
3. abdominal aorta above bifurcation
4. nerve rootlets of cauda equina in thecal sac
5. L4 nerve rootlet bundle in thecal sac
6. L3 nerve root
7. erector spinae muscle group
8. lamina L3
9. spinous process L3
10. ligamentum flavum
11. multifidis muscle
12. facet joint L3-4
13. quadratus lumborum muscle
14. psoas muscle

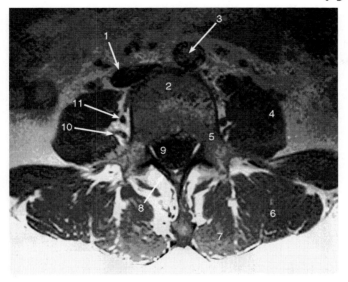

FIG. 63. Axial T1 spin echo: L4 vertebral body level
1. inferior vena cava
2. L4 vertebral body
3. abdominal aorta
4. psoas muscle
5. pedicle L4
6. erector spinae muscle group
7. multifidis muscle
8. lamina L4
9. subarachnoid space
10. L3 nerve root, ventral ramus
11. paravertebral longitudinal vein

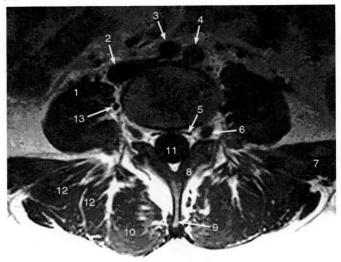

FIG. 64. Axial T1 spin echo: Upper L4-5 foramen
1. psoas muscle
2. inferior vena cava
3. right common iliac artery
4. left common iliac artery
5. anterior epidural veins
6. dorsal root ganglion L4
7. quadratus lumborum muscle
8. lamina L4
9. spinous process L4
10. multifidis muscle
11. subarachnoid space
12. erector spinae muscle group
13. paravertebral longitudinal vein

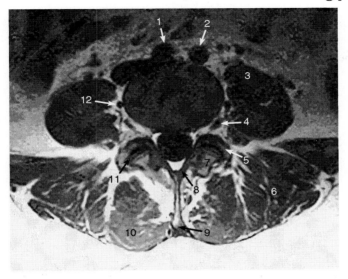

FIG. 65. Axial T1 spin echo: Low L4-5 foramen level
1. right common iliac artery
2. left common iliac artery
3. psoas muscle
4. L4 nerve root, ventral ramus
5. superior articular facet L5
6. erector spinae muscle group
7. inferior articular process L4
8. ligamentum flavum
9. spinous process L4
10. multifidis muscle
11. facet joint L4-5
12. paravertebral longitudinal vein

Lumbar Spine

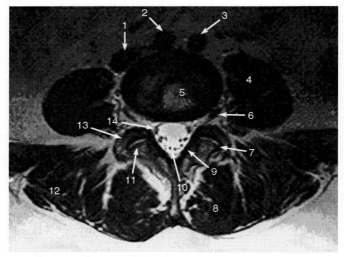

FIG. 66. Axial T2 fast spin echo: L4-5 disc level
1. inferior vena cava
2. right common iliac artery
3. left common iliac artery
4. psoas muscle
5. L4-5 intervertebral disc
6. L4 nerve root
7. facet joint L4-5
8. multifidis muscle
9. ligamentum flavum
10. nerve rootlets of cauda equina in thecal sac
11. inferior articular process L4
12. erector spinae muscle group
13. superior articular process L5
14. L5 nerve rootlets in thecal sac

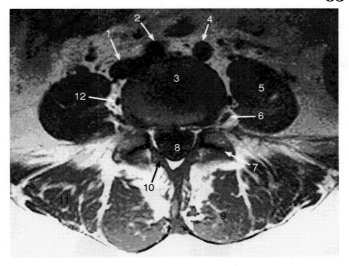

FIG. 67. Axial T1 spin echo: L4-5 intervertebral disc
1. inferior vena cava
2. right common iliac artery
3. L4-5 intervertebral disc
4. left common iliac artery
5. psoas muscle
6. L4 nerve root, ventral ramus
7. L4-5 facet joint
8. subarachnoid space
9. multifidis muscle
10. ligamentum flavum
11. erector spinae muscle group
12. paravertebral longitudinal vein

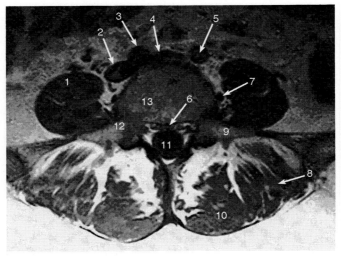

FIG. 68. Axial T1 spin echo: L5 vertebral body level
1. psoas muscle
2. right common iliac vein
3. right common iliac artery
4. left common iliac vein
5. left common iliac artery
6. anterior epidural venous plexus
7. paravertebral longitudinal vein
8. erector spinae muscle group
9. transverse process L5
10. multifidis muscle
11. subarachnoid space
12. pedicle L5
13. L5 vertebral body

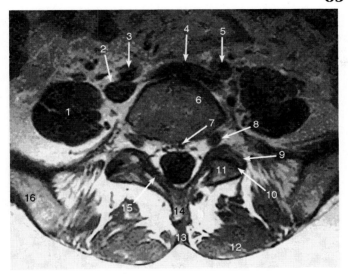

FIG. 69. Axial T1 spin echo: Upper L5-S1 foramen level
1. psoas muscle
2. right common iliac vein
3. right common iliac artery
4. left common iliac vein
5. left common iliac artery
6. L5 vertebral body
7. anterior epidural venous plexus
8. L5 dorsal root ganglion
9. superior articular process S1
10. facet joint L5-S1
11. inferior articular process L5
12. multifidis muscle
13. supraspinous ligament
14. spinous process L5
15. ligamentum flavum
16. iliac bone

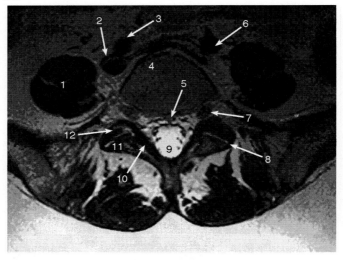

FIG. 70. Axial T2 fast spin echo: Upper L5-S1 foramen level

1. psoas muscle
2. right common iliac vein
3. right common iliac artery
4. L5 vertebral body
5. anterior epidural veins
6. left common iliac artery
7. dorsal root ganglion L5
8. facet joint L5-S1
9. subarachnoid space containing nerve rootlets
10. ligamentum flavum
11. inferior articular process L5
12. superior articular process S1

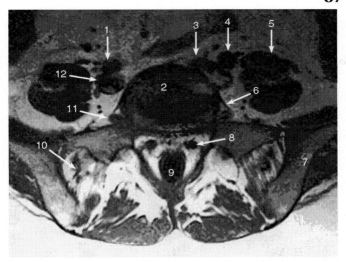

FIG. 71. Axial T1 spin echo: L5-S1 disc level
1. right common iliac artery
2. L5-S1 intervertebral disc
3. left common iliac vein
4. left common iliac artery
5. psoas muscle
6. iliolumbar ligament
7. iliac bone
8. S1 nerve root/sheath
9. subarachnoid space
10. sacroiliac joint, superior fibrous portion
11. L5 nerve root, ventral ramus (just above lumbosacral trunk)
12. right common iliac vein

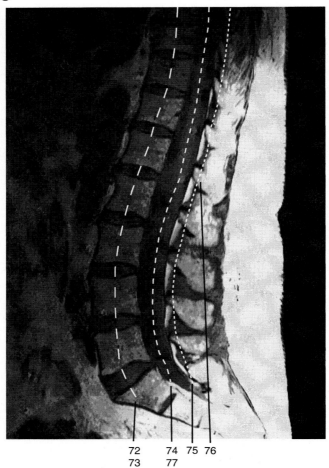

72 74 75 76
73 77

(L12) Localizer for coronal lumbar spine images.

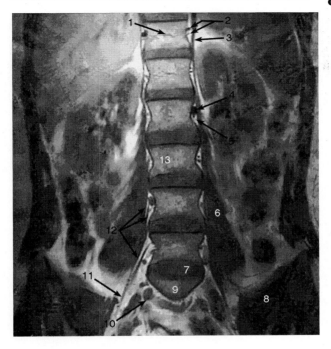

FIG. 72. Coronal T1 curved reformatted spin echo through lumbar vertebral bodies
1. basivertebral vein, vertebral body centrum
2. T11 intercostal vein (above) and intercostal artery (below)
3. crus of diaphragm
4. L1 lumbar paravertebral vein
5. L1 lumbar artery
6. psoas muscle
7. L5-S1 intervertebral disc
8. iliacus muscle
9. L5 vertebral body
10. L5 dorsal root ganglion
11. lumbosacral trunk
12. lumbar neural plexus
13. L2 vertebral body

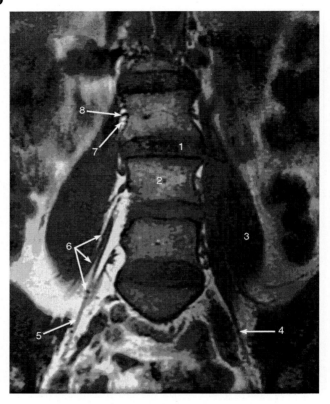

FIG. 73. Coronal curved reformatted T1 spin echo of the lumbar spine: Magnified view of lumbar neural plexus
1. intervertebral disc
2. vertebral body
3. psoas muscle
4. left lumbosacral trunk
5. right lumbosacral trunk
6. lumbar neural plexus (formed from ventral rami)
7. lumbar artery
8. lumbar vein

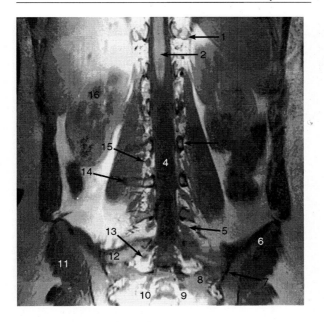

FIG. 74. Coronal T1 spin echo curved reformatted through spinal canal
1. head of T11 rib
2. conus medullaris
3. L2 pedicle
4. subarachnoid space
5. L4 dorsal root ganglion
6. iliac crest
7. sacroiliac joint
8. sacral wing
9. left S1 nerve root
10. right S1 nerve root
11. gluteus muscles
12. sacralized L5 vertebral segment
13. L5 dorsal root ganglion
14. transverse process L3
15. dorsal root ganglion L2
16. right kidney

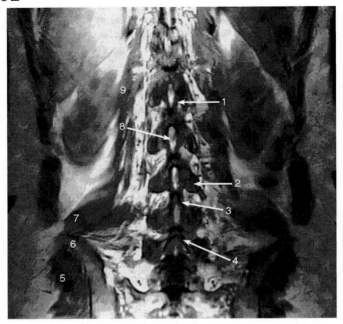

FIG. 75. Curved reformatted coronal T1 spin echo: Ligamentum flavum/lamina
1. ligamentum flavum
2. facet joint
3. base of spinous process
4. lamina
5. gluteus muscle group
6. iliac crest
7. quadratus lumborum muscle
8. posterior epidural fat
9. psoas muscle

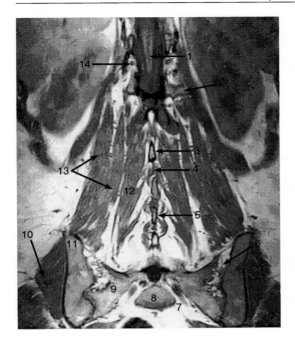

FIG. 76. Coronal T1 spin echo through spinous processes, paraspinal muscles
1. conus medullaris
2. transverse process
3. spinous process L2
4. interspinalis lumborum muscle
5. spinous process L4
6. sacroiliac joint, fibrous portion
7. S1 nerve root in 1st sacral neural foramen
8. S2 vertebral body
9. sacral wing
10. gluteus muscles
11. iliac crest
12. multifidis muscle
13. erector spinae muscle group
14. dorsal root ganglion

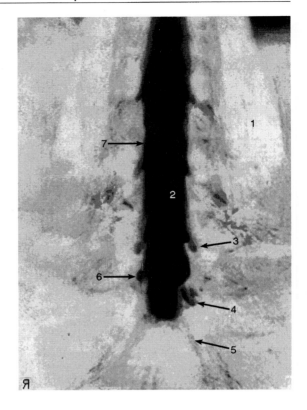

FIG. 77. MR "myelogram": Composite AP view from coronal data set
1. psoas muscle
2. subarachnoid space
3. nerve root and sleeve L5
4. nerve root and sleeve S1
5. nerve root S2
6. nerve root pouch S1
7. thecal sac margin

Sacrum _____

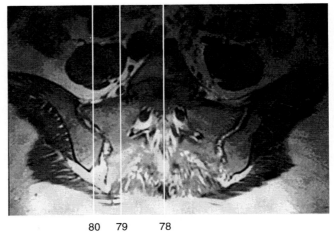

80   79   78

(L13) Localizer for sagittal images of sacrum.

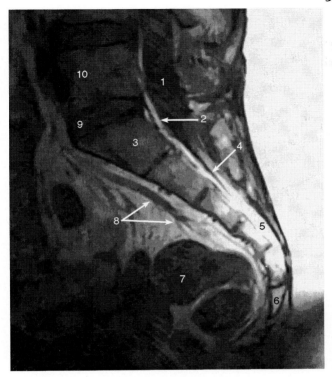

FIG. 78. Midsagittal T1 spine echo: Sacral spinal canal
 1. subarachnoid space
 2. ventral epidural space
 3. vertebral body S1
 4. filum terminale/caudal dura
 5. caudal epidural fat in sacral spinal canal
 6. 1st coccygeal vertebral segment
 7. rectosigmoid colon
 8. presacral vessels
 9. intervertebral disc L5-S1
10. vertebral body L5

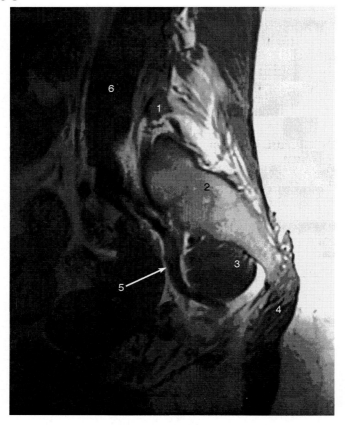

FIG. 79. Parasagittal T1 spine echo: Sacral wing
1. transverse process L5
2. sacral wing
3. bowel
4. gluteus maximus muscle
5. right internal Iliac vein
6. abdominal aorta

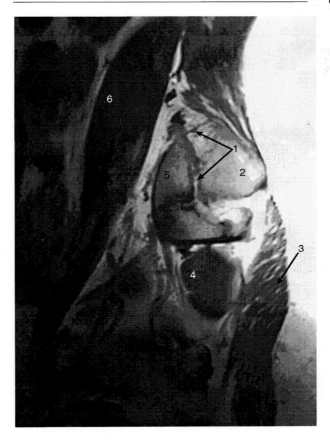

FIG. 80. Parasagittal T1 spin echo: Sacroiliac joint
1. sacroiliac joint
2. iliac bone
3. gluteus maximus muscle
4. bowel
5. sacrum
6. psoas muscle

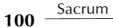

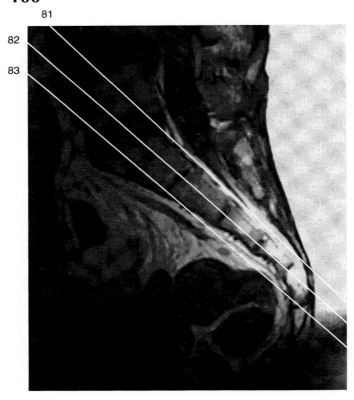

(L14) Localizer for oblique coronal images of sacrum.

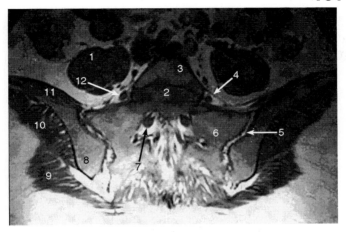

FIG. 81. Oblique coronal T1 spin echo: Sacral spinal canal

1. psoas muscle
2. intervertebral disc L5-S1
3. vertebral body L5
4. iliolumbar ligament
5. sacroiliac joint
6. sacral wing
7. S1 nerve root
8. iliac bone
9. gluteus maximus muscle
10. gluteus medius muscle
11. iliacus muscle
12. lumbosacral trunk

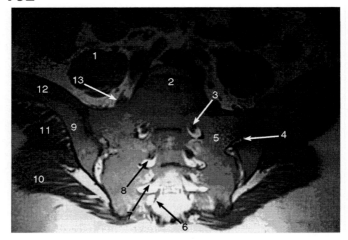

FIG. 82. Oblique coronal T1 spin echo: Sacral neural foramen
1. psoas muscle
2. intervertebral disc L5-S1
3. S1 nerve root
4. sacroiliac joint
5. sacral wing
6. S4 nerve root
7. S3 nerve root
8. S2 nerve root
9. iliac bone
10. gluteus maximus muscle
11. gluteus medius muscle
12. iliacus muscle
13. lumbosacral trunk

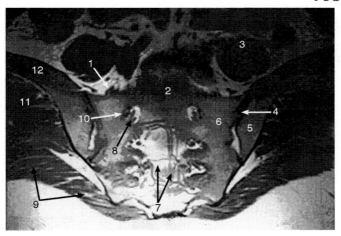

FIG. 83. Oblique coronal T1 spin echo: Ventral sacrum
1. lumbosacral trunk
2. S1 sacral segment
3. psoas muscle
4. sacroiliac joint
5. iliac bone
6. sacral wing
7. presacral vessels, mainly veins
8. nerve root S1
9. gluteus maximus muscle
10. foraminal vein S1
11. gluteus medius muscle
12. iliacus muscle

References

1. Koritke JG, Sick, H. *Atlas of Sectional Human Anatomy*, 2nd ed. Baltimore-Munich:Urban & Schwarzenberg, 1988.
2. Daniels DL, Haughton VM, Naidich T. *Cranial and Spinal Magnetic Resonance Imaging*. New York:Raven Press, 1987.
3. LaMasters DL, deGroot J. Normal craniocervical junction. In: *Computed Tomography of the Spine and Spinal Cord*. Newton TH, Potts DG, eds. San Anselmo, CA:Clavadel Press, 1983.
4. Czervionke LF, Daniels DL, Ho PSP, et al. The MR appearance of gray and white matter in the spinal cord. *Am J Neuroradiology* 1988;9:557–562.
5. Schnitzlein HN, Murtagh FR. *Imaging Anatomy of the Head and Spine*, 2nd ed. Baltimore-Munich:Urban & Schwarzenberg, 1990.
6. Eycleshymer AC, Schoemaker DM. *A Cross-Section Anatomy*. New York:Appleton-Century-Crofts, 1970.